CARNIVORE COOKBOOK

51 Delicious Beef, Pork and Buffalo Recipes, Easy to Cook from the Comfort of Your Home

Jason Pot

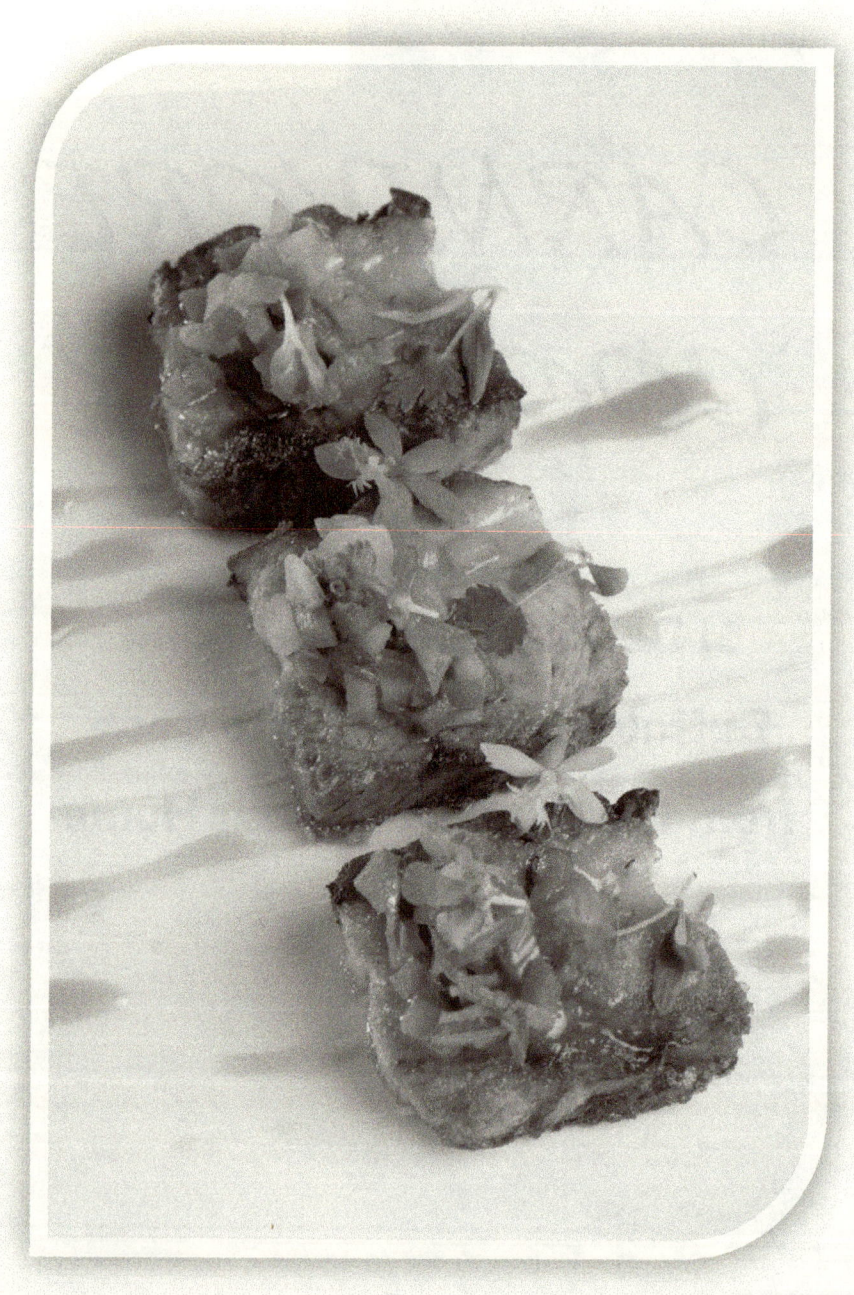

© **Copyright 2021 by Jason Pot - All rights reserved.**

The following Book is reproduced below with the goal of providing information that is as accurate and reliable as possible. Regardless, purchasing this Book can be seen as consent to the fact that both the publisher and the author of this book are in no way experts on the topics discussed within and that any recommendations or suggestions that are made herein are for entertainment purposes only. Professionals should be consulted as needed prior to undertaking any of the action endorsed herein.

This declaration is deemed fair and valid by both the American Bar Association and the Committee of Publishers Association and is legally binding throughout the United States.

Furthermore, the transmission, duplication, or reproduction of any of the following work including specific information will be considered an illegal act irrespective of if it is done electronically or in print. This extends to creating a secondary or tertiary copy of the work or a recorded copy and is only allowed with the express written consent from the Publisher. All additional right reserved.

The information in the following pages is broadly considered a truthful and accurate account of facts and as such, any inattention, use, or misuse of the information in question by the reader will render any resulting actions solely under their purview. There are no scenarios in which the publisher or the original author of this work can be in any fashion deemed liable for any hardship or damages that may befall them after undertaking information described herein.

Additionally, the information in the following pages is intended only for informational purposes and should thus be thought of as universal. As befitting its nature, it is presented without assurance regarding its prolonged validity or interim quality. Trademarks that are mentioned are done without written consent and can in no way be considered an endorsement from the trademark holder.

Table of Contents

1. Pork Medallions 7
2. Slow-Cooked Pork, Cider & Sage Hotpot 9
3. Pork Souvlaki 12
4. Beef Goulash 14
5. Pork Chops & Mustardy Butter Beans 16
6. Tonkatsu Pork 18
7. Pork Wellington 20
8. Pork Belly with Bay, Cider & Pears 24
9. Seared Beef Salad with Capers & Mint 27
10. Barbacoa Beef Tacos with Pickled Watermelon & Avocado Sauce ... 29
11. Balsamic Beef with Beetroot & Rocket 33
12. Italian-Style Beef Stew 35
13. Buffalo Wild Wings Grilled Chicken Wraps 37
14. Buffalo Wings Boneless Wings 39
15. Meat Loaf 41
16. Roast Beef 43
17. Grilled Pork Chops 45
18. Peppered Ribeye Steaks 47
19. Mushroom Braised Pot Roast 49
20. Shepherd's Pie 51
21. Steak Diane 53
22. Grilled Steak Medallions 55
23. Provolone Stuffed Meatballs 57
24. Brunch Burger 60
25. Quesadilla Burger 62
26. Honey Barbecue Riblets 66
27. Cilantro Beef Curry 69
28. Coconut Ribs Curry 71
29. Creamy Coconut Pork 73
30. Madras Tomato Beef 75
31. Ginger Beef Curry 77
32. Beef with Cardamom Veggies 79
33. Onion Beef in Yogurt 81
34. Ginger Beef Mix 83
35. Beef and Lentils Curry 85
36. Curry Pork with Lentils 87
37. Ground Beef Masala 89
38. Chili Beef and Peas 91
39. Coconut Masala Beef 93

40.	GRILLED STEAK SALAD WITH BLUE CHEESE DRESSING	95
41.	FILET MIGNON WITH PINEAPPLE SALSA	97
42.	CHILI-RUBBED FLANK STEAK	100
43.	SOY AND GARLIC STEAK KEBABS	102
44.	BEEF BULGOGI	104
45.	GOCHUJANG-MARINATED BABY BACK RIBS	106
46.	CHILI'S BONELESS BUFFALO WINGS	108
47.	CRUNCHY PORK WONTONS	110
48.	BUFFALO CHICKEN & BLUE CHEESE SLAW	112
49.	BAKED BUFFALO CHICKEN WINGS	114
50.	BUFFALO CAULIFLOWER	116
51.	PINEAPPLE & PORK SKEWERS	118

1. Pork Medallions

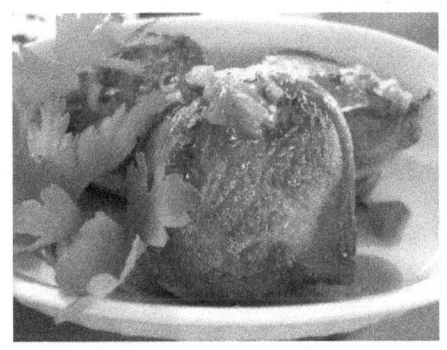

Preparation Time: 10 mins

Cooking Time: 30 mins

Easy

Serves: 4

Ingredients:

- 1 tbsp olive oil
- 600g pork medallions
- 2 tbsp unsalted butter
- 2 banana shallots, thinly sliced
- 250g chestnut mushrooms, sliced
- 1 garlic clove, crushed
- 1 tbsp plain flour
- 100ml madeira or sherry

- 400ml chicken stock
- 4 sprigs thyme
- ½ tbsp wholegrain mustard
- 100ml double cream
- mashed potato and wilted greens, to serve

Directions:

Heat the oil in a large non-stick frying pan and fry the pork on each side for 2-3 mins until golden brown. Set aside on a plate. Melt the butter in the pan and, when foaming, fry the shallots and mushrooms over a medium heat for 10 mins. Add the garlic and cook for another 1 min. Stir through the flour and cook for another 2 mins. Whisk through the madeira and boil for 2 mins. Gradually stir through the stock until the sauce is lump free. Add the thyme and mustard and season to taste. Return the pork to the pan and simmer uncovered for 5-7 mins or until the pork is cooked through. Stir through the cream and heat again until simmering. Serve with creamy mashed potatoes and wilted greens.

Nutrition:

Kcal 545, Fat: 40g, Saturates: 18g, Carbs: 7g, Sugars: 3g, Fibre: 2g, Protein: 31g, Salt: 0.9g

2. Slow-Cooked Pork, Cider & Sage Hotpot

Preparation Time: 40 mins
Cooking Time: 3 hrs
Serves: 6

Ingredients:

- 4 tbsp olive oil, plus a little extra
- 1kg diced pork shoulder
- 20g butter, cubed, plus a little extra
- 4 leeks, trimmed and thickly sliced
- 4 garlic cloves, crushed
- 3 tbsp plain flour
- 500ml dry cider
- 400ml chicken stock
- 2 bay leaves
- ½ small bunch parsley, finely chopped
- small bunch sage, leaves picked, 5 left whole, the rest chopped
- 200ml single cream
- 400g Maris Piper or King Edward potatoes
- 400g sweet potatoes

Directions:

Heat half of the oil in a deep ovenproof frying pan, or flameproof casserole dish, and fry the pork pieces over a medium high heat in batches until seared all over, then transfer to a plate. Add another 1 tbsp oil to the pan, if you need to, while you're cooking the batches. Once all the pork is seared, transfer to a plate and set aside. Add another 1 tbsp oil to the pan with a little butter and fry half the leeks with a pinch of salt for 10 mins until tender. Add the garlic, fry for a minute, then stir in the flour.

Pour in the cider, a little at a time, stirring to pick up any bits stuck to the bottom of the pan and to combine everything. Add the stock, bay leaves and seared pork, then simmer, half-covered with a lid for 1-1½ hrs until the meat is just tender (it will later cook to the point of falling apart in the oven). Can be prepared a day ahead.

Heat the oven to 200C/180C fan/gas 6.

Simmer uncovered for a few minutes to reduce the sauce, if you need to – it shouldn't be too liquid or the potatoes will sink into the sauce.

Stir in the parsley, chopped sage, remaining leeks, and the cream, then season well.

Peel both types of potatoes and cut into slices 2mm thick, by hand or using a mandoline. Alternate layers of potato and sweet potato in circles over the pie, or randomly, if you prefer. Dot the cubed butter over the top and bake for 1-1½ hrs until the potato is tender. Nestle in the whole sage leaves, brushed in a little oil, for the last 10 mins. Leave to rest for 10 mins before serving.

Nutrition:

Kcal 644, Fat: 35g, Saturates: 14g, Carbs: 39g, Sugars: 13g, Fibre: 80g, Protein: 35g, Salt: 0.6g

3. Pork Souvlaki

Preparation Time: 15 mins

Cooking Time: 10 mins plus marinating

Easy

Serves: 4

Ingredients:

- 400g lean pork shoulder, cut into 2cm chunks
- 1 tbsp olive oil
- ½ tbsp dried oregano
- 1 lemon , zested and juiced
- ½ tsp hot paprika
- 100ml fat-free yogurt
- 1 small garlic clove , grated
- ½ cucumber , trimmed and grated
- 2 red peppers , deseeded and cut into chunks
- 2 Little Gem lettuce , leaves separated
- chilli sauce , to serve (optional)
- flatbreads , warmed, to serve (optional)

Directions:

Put the pork in a large bowl with the oil, oregano, lemon zest and juice and paprika as well as a good pinch of salt. Toss everything together to combine and leave to marinate for 10 mins.

Combine the yogurt, garlic and cucumber together in a bowl. Season with salt and set aside.

Heat the grill to high. Thread the marinated pork and the peppers on four metal skewers, alternating between the pork and peppers as you go. Place on a non-stick baking sheet and grill for 3-4 mins on each side, or until cooked through and golden brown. Serve with the lettuce, yogurt mixture and chilli sauce, and flatbreads, if you like.

Nutrition:

Kcal 210, Fat: 8g, Saturates: 2g, Carbs: 8g, Sugars: 8g, Fibre: 5g, Protein: 25g, Salt: 0.3g

4. Beef Goulash

Preparation Time: 20 mins

Cooking Time: 2 hrs - 2 hrs and 30 mins

Easy

Serves: 4

Ingredients:

- 4 tbsp olive oil
- 700g stewing steak, cut into chunks
- 30g plain flour
- 1 large onion, thinly sliced
- 2 garlic cloves, finely chopped
- 1 green pepper, deseeded and thinly sliced
- 1 red pepper, deseeded and thinly sliced
- 2 tbsp tomato purée
- 2 tbsp paprika
- 2 large tomatoes, diced
- 75ml dry white wine
- 300ml beef stock, homemade or shop-bought
- 2 tbsp flat-leaf parsley leaves
- 150ml soured cream

Directions:

Heat oven to 160C/140C fan/gas 3.

Heat 1 tbsp olive oil in a flameproof casserole dish or heavy-based saucepan. Sprinkle 700g stewing steak chunks with 30g plain flour and brown well in three batches, adding an extra 1 tbsp oil for each batch. Set the browned meat aside. Add in the remaining 1 tbsp oil to the casserole dish, followed by 1 large thinly sliced onion, 2 finely chopped garlic cloves, 1 green pepper and 1 red pepper, both finely sliced. Fry until softened, around 5-10 mins. Return the beef to the pan with 2 tbsp tomato purée and 2 tbsp paprika. Cook, stirring, for 2 mins. Add in 2 large diced tomatoes, 75ml dry white wine and 300ml beef stock. Cover and bake in the oven for 1 hr 30 mins - 2 hrs. Alternatively, cover and cook it on the hob on a gentle heat for about an hour, removing the lid after 45 mins. Sprinkle over 2 tbsp flat-leaf parsley leaves and season well with salt and freshly ground pepper. Stir in 150ml soured cream and serve.

Nutrition:

Kcal 576, Fat: 32g, Saturates: 12g, Carbs: 18g, Sugars: 11g, Fibre: 6g, Protein: 46g, Salt: 0.45g

5. Pork Chops & Mustardy Butter Beans

Preparation Time: 10 mins

Cooking Time: 30 mins

Easy

Serves: 2

Ingredients:

- 2 tbsp olive oil
- 1 onion , finely sliced
- 1 small garlic clove , crushed
- 400g can butter beans , drained and rinsed
- 100ml chicken stock
- 200g spinach
- 3 tbsp crème fraîche
- ½ tbsp wholegrain mustard
- 2 pork chops

Directions:

Heat 1 tbsp of the oil in a saucepan. Add the onion and fry over a medium heat for 10 mins, or until softened. Add the garlic and cook for 1 min.

Stir through the butter beans and stock and bring to a simmer. Add the spinach. Cover and cook for 3 mins or until the spinach is wilted.

Blitz the mixture using a hand blender for 10 secs, leaving some chunky, whole beans. Stir through the crème fraîche and mustard and season generously, then simmer for 3 mins to thicken. Set aside.

Season the pork chops on both sides. Heat the remaining oil in a non-stick pan over a medium-high heat. Hold the chops on their sides with a pair of tongs to brown the fat. Cook each one on either side for 7 mins or until cooked through. Spoon the beans onto plates, slice the pork and arrange on top.

Nutrition:
Kcal 610, Fat: 37g, Saturates: 12g, Carbs: 22g, Sugars: 7g, Fibre: 9g, Protein: 43g, Salt: 0.8g

6. Tonkatsu Pork

Preparation Time: 20 mins
Cooking Time: 6 mins

 **Easy**

Serves: 4

Ingredients:

- 4 thick boneless pork loin chops
- 100g plain flour
- 2 eggs , beaten
- 100g panko breadcrumbs
- vegetable oil , for shallow frying

For the sauce:

- 2 tbsp ketchup
- 2 tbsp Worcestershire sauce
- 1 tbsp oyster sauce
- 2 tsp caster sugar

Directions:

Remove the large piece of fat on the edge of each pork loin, then bash each of the loins between two pieces of baking parchment until around 1cm in thickness – you can do this using a meat tenderiser or a rolling pin. Once bashed, use your hands to reshape the meat to its original shape and thickness – this step will ensure the meat is as succulent as possible. Put the flour, eggs and panko breadcrumbs into three separate wide-rimmed bowls. Season the meat, then dip first in the flour, followed by the eggs, then the breadcrumbs.

In a large frying or sauté pan, add enough oil to come 2cm up the side of the pan. Heat the oil to 180C – if you don't have a thermometer, drop a bit of panko into the oil and if it sinks a little then starts to fry, the oil is ready. Add two pork chops and cook for 1 min 30 secs on each side, then remove and leave to rest on a wire rack for 5 mins. Repeat with the remaining pork chops. While the pork is resting, make the sauce by whisking the ingredients together, adding a splash of water if it's particularly thick. Slice the tonkatsu and serve drizzled with the sauce.

Nutrition:

Kcal 576,   Fat: 25g,   Saturates: 8g,   Carbs: 43g,   Sugars: 6g,   Fibre: 2g,   Protein: 42g,   Salt: 1.5g

7. Pork Wellington

Preparation Time: 45 mins

Cooking Time: 1 hr plus chilling

Serves: 6 – 8

Ingredients:

- olive oil , for frying
- 2 large pork fillets (approx 800g), trimmed and the ends removed
- 1 shallot , finely chopped
- 50g butter
- 150g wild mushrooms (such as chanterelles), finely chopped
- handful sage , picked and chopped
- handful parsley , chopped
- good handful chives , snipped
- 100g spinach
- 10 slices prosciutto
- 50g good-quality chicken liver pâté

For the pastry:

- 500g pack puff pastry
- plain flour , for dusting

- 2 egg yolks , beaten with 1 tsp water

For the mustard:
- 300ml pot double cream
- 3 tbsp Dijon mustard

Directions:

Heat a pan with a little oil to a very high heat and season the pork fillets well all over. Put 1 fillet in the pan and fry for 2 mins to give it a little colour all over. Remove and repeat with the other fillet, then leave both to rest and cool. Fry the shallot in the butter in the same pan for 2 mins, then add the mushrooms and cook until both are soft. Add the herbs and cook for 1 min. Season, tip 1/ 3 of the mixture into one bowl (reserved for the sauce) and the rest into another, and set aside to cool. Don't wash the pan. Meanwhile, heat a little oil in another large pan, add the spinach and cook briefly until wilted. Set aside until cool enough to squeeze out all the excess moisture, then chop. Tip the spinach into the first pan and use it to wipe up all the seasoning and juices. Overlap two pieces of cling film over a large chopping board. Lay the slices of prosciutto on the cling film in two rows, slightly overlapping.

Carefully spread the pâté mixture over the prosciutto, then sit the pork fillets on top. Pack the mushrooms in the gaps, then top with the spinach. Use the cling film to draw the prosciutto around the fillet mixture, then roll it into a sausage shape, twisting the ends of cling film to tighten it as you go. Chill while you roll out the pastry. Dust the work surface with a little flour. Roll out a third of the pastry to an 18 x 30cm strip about 2mm thick and place on a non-stick baking sheet. Roll out the remainder of the pastry to about 28 x 36cm, also 2mm thick. Unroll the fillet from the cling film and sit it in the centre of the smaller strip of pastry. Brush the pastry's edges with the yolk mixture, as well as the top and sides of the wrapped fillet. Using a rolling pin, lift and drape the larger piece of pastry over the fillet, pressing well into the sides. Trim the joins to about a 4cm rim. Seal the rim with the edge of a spoon handle. Glaze all over with more egg yolk and, if you like, mark the wellington using the back of a knife, taking care not to cut into the pastry. Chill for at least 30 mins or up to 24 hrs.

6 Heat oven to 200C/180C fan/gas 6. Brush the wellington with a little more egg yolk and cook for 35-40 mins until golden – the pork will be just pink in the middle. Allow to stand for 10 mins before serving in thick slices.

To make the sauce, bring the cream to the boil, add the mustard and reserved mushroom mixture, and remove from the heat. Season and stir well before serving.

Nutrition: per serving (8)
Kcal 709, Fat: 53g, Saturates: 27g, Carbs: 22g, Sugars: 2g, Fibre: 2g, Protein: 33g, Salt: 2.2g

8. Pork Belly with Bay, Cider & Pears

Preparation Time: 15 mins

Cooking Time: 2 hrs plus 4 hrs curing and resting

Easy

Serves: 6

Ingredients:

- 1½kg pork belly, skin scored
- rapeseed oil, for drizzling
- 1 carrot, roughly chopped
- 1 celery stick, roughly chopped
- 1 white onion or 4 shallots, roughly chopped
- 1 star anise
- 3 bay leaves
- 2 pears, cored and quartered
- 200ml dry pear cider
- 1 tbsp plain flour
- roast potatoes and steamed greens, to serve (optional)

For the rub:
- 3 tsp sea salt flakes
- 1 tsp fennel seeds
- 1 tsp white peppercorns

Directions:

To make the rub, put the ingredients in a pestle and mortar and crush together. Reserve ½ tsp of the rub and set aside. Cut some slashes into the underside of the pork using a sharp knife, then pat the rub all over the flesh, avoiding the skin. Put on a plate, skin-side up, and leave to cure in the fridge for at least 3 hrs. Remove the pork from the fridge at least 30 mins before cooking so it comes to room temperature. Heat the oven to 180C/160C fan/gas 4. Pat the reserved rub over the pork skin, and rub a little rapeseed oil all over. Put the carrot, celery, onion, star anise and bay leaves in a large flameproof roasting tin. Pour over a small glass of water, then place the pork on top, skin-side up. Roast for 1 hr 30 mins. Arrange the pears in the tin around the pork, coating them in the juices, and pour the cider into the tin, avoiding the pork skin (if the skin gets wet, you won't end up with crisp crackling). Turn the oven up to 220C/200C fan/gas 7 and roast for a further 15-20 mins. The pork skin should be crisp, and the pears glazed in the juices. Remove the pork from the tin. Leave to rest for 45 mins. Transfer the pork to a serving platter. Gently lift the pears out of the tin and arrange next to the pork. Discard the carrot, celery, onion and bay, then skim some of the fat from the surface of the juices (you can transfer this fat to a jar and use it for cooking roast potatoes, or making rillettes, and more).

Put the roasting tin with the skimmed juices on the hob over a medium heat. Sprinkle in the flour and whisk it into the juices until smooth and thickened. Add a splash of hot water if it becomes too thick. Pour the gravy into a warm jug. Cut the pork into portions with a sharp knife, then serve with the roasted pear quarters, the gravy, and some roast potatoes and steamed greens, if you like.

Nutrition:
Kcal 547,   Fat: 37g,   Saturates: 12g,   Carbs: 9g, Sugars: 6g,   Fibre: 2g,   Protein: 42g,   Salt: 2.8g

9. Seared Beef Salad with Capers & Mint

Preparation Time: 10 mins
Cooking Time: 12 mins

Easy

Serves: 2

Ingredients:

- 150g new potatoes, thickly sliced
- 160g fine green beans, trimmed and halved
- 160g frozen peas
- rapeseed oil, for brushing
- 200g lean fillet steak, trimmed of any fat
- 160g romaine lettuce, roughly torn into pieces

For the dressing:

- 1 tbsp extra virgin olive oil
- 2 tsp cider vinegar
- ½ tsp English mustard powder
- 2 tbsp chopped mint
- 3 tbsp chopped basil
- 1 garlic clove, finely grated

- 1 tbsp capers

Directions:

Cook the potatoes in a pan of simmering water for 5 mins. Add the beans and cook 5 mins more, then tip in the peas and cook for 2 mins until all the vegetables are just tender. Drain. Meanwhile, measure all the dressing ingredients in a large bowl and season with black pepper. Stir and crush the herbs and capers with the back of a spoon to intensify their flavours. Brush a little oil over the steak and grind over some black pepper. Heat a non-stick frying pan over a high heat and cook the steak for 4 mins on one side and 2-3 mins on the other, depending on the thickness and how rare you like it. Transfer to a plate to rest while you carry on with the rest of the salad. Mix the warm vegetables into the dressing until well coated, then add the lettuce and toss again. Pile onto plates. Slice the steak and turn in any dressing left in the bowl, add to the salad and serve while still warm.

Nutrition:

low in kcal:357, fat: 13g, saturates: 4g, salt: 0.5g carbs: 25g, sugars: 8g, fibre: 12g, protein: 29g,

10. Barbacoa Beef Tacos with Pickled Watermelon & Avocado Sauce

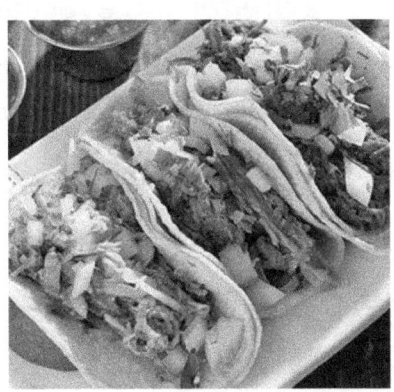

Preparation Time: 25 mins

Cooking Time: 5 hrs plus overnight marinating and 1 hr chilling

Serves: 8

Ingredients:
- 24 small corn tortillas , to serve

For the marinade:
- 2 red onions , cut into wedges
- 3 whole tomatoes
- 10 garlic cloves

- 2 ancho chillies
- 3 tbsp smoky Mexican spice mix , plus 1 tsp for the watermelon (see below)
- 75ml vegetable oil , plus 2 tbsp
- 2-3 lemons (2 are for the avocado cream)
- 2kg boneless beef brisket or blade, cut into chunks (ask your butcher to do this for you)
- 500ml chicken stock
- 3 bay leaves

For the avocado cream:
- 3 avocados
- 6 tbsp soured cream
- 1 small pack coriander , stems chopped, leaves kept whole

For the pickled watermelon:
- 50ml white wine vinegar
- 1 tsp sugar
- ½ small watermelon, cut into cubes, any large seeds removed

For the smoky Mexican spice mix:
- 1 tbsp cumin seeds
- 1½ tsp ground oregano
- 2 tsp smoked paprika

- 4 ground cloves
- 2 tbsp smoked salt flakes
- 2 tbsp chipotle chilli flakes

Directions:

The day before, make the marinade. Put the red onion, tomatoes and garlic cloves in a dry non-stick frying pan over a medium heat.

Fry, shaking the pan occasionally, until blackened – this will add flavour. Tip into a blender. Return the pan to the heat, add the chillies, toast until fragrant, then tip into the blender as well, along with 3 tbsp spice mix, 75ml oil and the juice of 1 lemon. Blitz until smooth. Pour a little of the leftover oil into the frying pan over a medium-high heat. Season, then brown the beef in batches until each piece has a nice dark brown crust. Tip the beef into a large, ovenproof dish with a lid, then pour over the marinade. Toss to coat, cover and chill in the fridge overnight. Heat oven to 150C/130C fan/gas 2.

Take the dish out the fridge.

Pour in the stock, add the bay leaves, then mix together.

Pop on the lid and cook for 3½ hrs, removing the lid for the last hour, until the meat falls apart when prodded. Remove the beef from the dish and set aside, then put the dish back on the heat and bubble until the sauce has reduced by half. Shred the beef with two forks and add back to the sauce.
Meanwhile, put the avocados, soured cream and coriander stalks in a blender.
Squeeze in the juice of 1 lemon. Blitz until smooth, then season and add more lemon juice to taste. Set aside in the fridge. For the pickled watermelon, whisk the vinegar, sugar and 1 tsp spice mix together in a bowl. Add the watermelon and toss to coat. Cover and chill for 1 hr, tossing occasionally, to lightly pickle. To serve, warm the tortillas in a frying pan. Spread some of the avocado cream on each one, top with a pile of beef, a few cubes of watermelon and some coriander.

Nutrition:
Kcal 770, Fat: 43g, Saturates: 13g, Carbs: 54g, Sugars: 12g, Fibre: 5g, Protein: 40g, Salt: 2.6g

11. Balsamic Beef with Beetroot & Rocket

 **Preparation Time:** 15 mins
Cooking Time: 25 mins

Easy

Serves: 2

Ingredients

- 240g beef sirloin , fat trimmed
- 1 tbsp balsamic vinegar
- 2 tsp thyme leaves
- 2 garlic cloves , 1 finely grated, 1 sliced
- 2 tsp rapeseed oil
- 2 red onions , halved and sliced
- 175g fine beans , trimmed
- 2 cooked beetroot, halved and cut into wedges
- 6 pitted Kalamata olives , quartered
- 2 handfuls rocket

Directions:

Beat the steak with a rolling pin until it is about the thickness of two £1 coins, then cut into two equal pieces. In a bowl, mix the balsamic, thyme, grated garlic, half the oil and a grinding of black pepper. Place the steaks in the marinade and set aside. Heat the remaining 1 tsp oil in a large non-stick frying pan, and fry the onions and garlic for 8-10 mins, stirring frequently, until soft and starting to brown. Meanwhile, steam the beans for 4-6 mins or until just tender.

Push the onion mixture to one side in the pan. Lift the steaks from the bowl, shake off any excess marinade, and sear in the pan for 2½-3 mins, turning once, until cooked but still a little pink inside. Pile the beans onto plates and place the steaks on top. Add the beetroot wedges, olives and remaining marinade to the pan and cook briefly to heat through, then spoon on top and around the steaks. Add the rocket and serve.

Nutrition:

low in kcal 284, fat: 9g, saturates: 3g, carbs: 19g, sugars: 15g, fibre: 9g, protein: 27g, salt: 0.6g

12. Italian-Style Beef Stew

Preparation Time: 10 minutes
Cooking Time: 20 mins

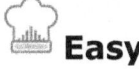**Easy**

Serves: 4

Ingredients:

- 1 onion, sliced
- 1 garlic clove, sliced
- 2 tbsp olive oil
- 300g pack beef stir-fry strips, or use beef steak, thinly sliced
- 1 yellow pepper, deseeded and thinly sliced
- 400g can chopped tomato
- sprig rosemary, chopped
- handful pitted olives

Directions:

In a large saucepan, cook onion and garlic in olive oil for 5 mins until softened and turning golden. Tip in the beef strips, pepper, tomatoes and rosemary, then bring to the boil. Simmer for 15 mins until the meat is cooked through, adding some boiling water if needed. Stir through the olives and serve with mash or polenta.

Nutrition:

Kcal 225, Fat: 11g, Saturates: 3g, Carbs: 7g, Sugars: 6g, Fibre: 2g, Protein: 25g, low in salt: 0.87g

13. Buffalo Wild Wings Grilled Chicken Wraps

Preparation time: 35 Minutes

Cooking time: 10 minutes

Servings: 4

Ingredients:

- 1 lb. boneless skinless chicken breasts
- 2 teaspoons vegetable oil
- 1 cup KRAFT Mexican Style cheese, shredded
- 1 tomato, chopped
- 3 tablespoons KRAFT Zesty Italian Dressing
- 2 teaspoons chili powder
- 4 (8") flour tortillas

Directions:

Heat grill to medium heat; Coat the chicken with oil and then grill for approximately 8 minutes per side or until done (165ºF); cool slightly; Cut the chicken into strips and place in a clean medium bowl; Add cheese, dressing, tomatoes, and chili powder; mix lightly; Spoon down centers of tortillas. Fold in opposing sides of tortillas, and then roll up burrito style; Place, seam sides down, on the grill grate. Grill 4-5 minutes per side or until evenly browned.

Nutrition:

Calorie: 570 kcal, Fat: 57 g, Carbs: 22 g, Sodium: 1560 mg, Protein: 4 g Potassium: 602mg, Fiber: 3g, Sugar: 3g

14. Buffalo Wings Boneless Wings

Preparation time: 10 minutes

Cooking time: 40 minutes

Servings: 4

Ingredients:

- Cooking Oil for deep frying
- 1 ⅓ cups unbleached flour, all-purpose
- 2 ¾ teaspoons salt
- ¾ teaspoon black pepper, ground
- ¾ teaspoon cayenne pepper
- ¼ teaspoon garlic powder, granulated
- ¾ teaspoon paprika
- 1 ¼ egg
- 1 ⅓ cups milk
- 4 skinless, boneless chicken breasts cut into ½" strips
- ⅓ cup hot pepper sauce
- 1 tablespoon
- 1 teaspoon butter

Directions:

Add and preheat oil in a large-sized saucepan or a deep fryer to 375° F; Combine paprika, garlic powder, cayenne pepper, salt, black pepper, and flour in a big bowl; Whisk together the egg as well as milk in a clean small bowl; Dip each piece of chicken in the egg mixture and then roll in the flour blend. Repeat so that each slice of chicken is double-coated; Refrigerate breaded chicken for twenty minutes; Fry the chicken in batches in the hot oil. Cook until the outside is nicely browned, as well as the juices runs clear, 5 to 6 minutes a batch; Combine sauce that is hot as well as butter in a clean small bowl; Microwave sauce on High until melted, 5-6 seconds; Pour sauce over the prepared chicken; Mix to coat.

Nutrition:

Calorie: 850 kcal, Fat: 52 g, Carbs: 58 g, Sodium: 2430 mg, Protein: 37 g

15. Meat Loaf

Preparation Time: 15 minutes

Cooking Time: 1 ½ hours

Servings: 6

Ingredients:

- 2 large eggs
- 2/3 cup whole milk
- 3 slices bread, torn
- 1/2 cup chopped onion
- 1/2 cup grated carrot
- 1 cup shredded cheddar or part-skim mozzarella cheese
- 1 tablespoon minced fresh parsley or 1 teaspoon dried parsley
- 1 teaspoon dried basil, thyme, or sage, optional 1 teaspoon salt 1/4 teaspoon pepper
- 1-1/2 pounds lean ground beef

Topping:

- 1/2 cup tomato sauce
- 1/2 cup packed brown sugar
- 1 teaspoon prepared mustard

Directions:

In a large bowl, beat eggs. Add milk and bread; let stand until liquid is absorbed. Stir in the onion, carrot, cheese, and seasonings. Crumble beef over mixture and mix well. Shape into a 7-1/2x3-1/2x2-1/2-in. loaf in a shallow baking pan. Bake, uncovered, at 350° for 45 minutes. Combine the topping ingredients, spoon half of the mixture over meat loaf. Bake 30 minutes longer or until meat is no longer pink and a thermometer reads 160°, occasionally spooning remaining topping over loaf. Let stand 10 minutes before serving.

Nutrition:

Calories: 398, Fat: 17g, Saturated fat: 9g, Cholesterol: 164mg, Sodium: 771mg, Protein: 30g, Carbohydrate: 29g, Sugar: 22g, Fiber: 1g,

16. Roast Beef

Preparation Time: 20 minutes

Cooking Time: 2 ½ hours

Servings: 8

Ingredients:

- 1 tablespoon canola oil
- 1 beef eye round roast (about 2-1/2 pounds)
- 1 garlic clove, minced
- 2 teaspoons dried basil
- 1 teaspoon salt
- 1 teaspoon dried rosemary, crushed
- 1/2 teaspoon pepper
- 1 medium onion, chopped
- 1 teaspoon beef bouillon granules
- 1 cup brewed coffee
- 3/4 cup water

Gravy:

- 1/4 cup all-purpose flour
- 1/4 cup cold water

Directions:

In a Dutch oven, heat oil over medium heat; brown roast on all sides. Remove from pan. Mix garlic and seasonings, sprinkle over roast. Add onion to same pan; cook and stir over medium heat until tender; stir in bouillon, coffee and 3/4 cup water. Add roast; bring to a boil. Reduce heat; simmer, covered, until meat is tender, about 2-1/2 hours. Remove roast from pan, reserving cooking juices. Tent with foil; let stand 10 minutes before slicing. Mix flour and cold water until smooth; stir into cooking juices. Bring to a boil, stirring constantly.

Cook and stir until thickened, 1-2 minutes. Serve with roast.

Nutrition:

Calories: 198, Fat: 6g, Protein: 28g
Cholesterol:65mg, Sodium:453mg, Carbohydrate: 5g

17. Grilled Pork Chops

Preparation Time: 20 minutes

Cooking Time: 10 minutes

Servings: 4

Ingredients:

- 1/4 cup kosher salt
- 1/4 cup sugar
- 2 cups water
- 2 cups ice water
- 4 center-cut pork rib chops (1 inch thick and 8 ounces each)
- 2 tablespoons canola oil

Basic Rub:

- 3 tablespoons paprika
- 1 teaspoon each garlic powder, onion powder, ground cumin and ground mustard
- 1 teaspoon coarsely ground pepper
- 1/2 teaspoon ground chipotle pepper

Directions:

In a large saucepan, combine salt, sugar and 2 cups water; cook and stir over medium heat until salt and sugar are dissolved. Remove from heat. Add 2 cups ice water to cool brine to room temperature. Place pork chops in a large resealable plastic bag; add cooled brine. Seal bag, pressing out as much air as possible; turn to coat chops. Place in a 13x9-in. baking dish. Refrigerate 8-12 hours. Remove chops from brine, rinse, and pat dry. Discard brine. Brush both sides of chops with oil. In a small bowl, mix rub ingredients; rub over pork chops. Let stand at room temperature 30 minutes. Grill chops on an oiled rack, covered, over medium heat 4-6 minutes on each side or until a thermometer reads 145°. Let stand 5 minutes before serving.

Nutrition:
Calories: 300, Cholesterol: 72mg, Fat: 18g Sodium: 130mg, Carbohydrate: 5g, Protein: 30g

18. Peppered Ribeye Steaks

Preparation Time: 10 minutes
Cooking Time: 10 minutes
Servings: 8

Ingredients:

- 1 tablespoon garlic powder
- 1 tablespoon paprika
- 2 teaspoons dried ground thyme
- 2 teaspoons dried ground oregano
- 1-1/2 teaspoons kosher salt
- 1-1/2 teaspoons pepper
- 1 teaspoon lemon-pepper seasoning
- 1 teaspoon cayenne pepper
- 1 teaspoon crushed red pepper flakes
- 4 beef ribeye steaks (1-1/2 inches thick and 8 ounces each)

Directions:

Combine all seasonings. Sprinkle over steaks, pressing mixture into both sides to help it adhere. Refrigerate, covered, for at least 1 hour or up to 24 hours. Remove steaks; blot with paper towels to remove any surface moisture, taking care to leave as much garlic mixture on steaks as possible. If desired, sprinkle with additional kosher salt. Grill steaks, covered, turning occasionally, on a greased grill rack over medium indirect heat until a thermometer reads 110°. Move steaks to direct heat; continue grilling until meat reaches desired doneness (for medium-rare, a thermometer should read 135°; medium, 140°; medium-well, 145°). Let stand 5 minutes before slicing. Place on a warm serving platter; cut across grain into thick slices.

Nutrition:

Calories: 257,   Cholesterol: 67mg,   Fat: 18g
Sodium: 453mg, Carbohydrate: 2g,   Protein: 21g,

19. Mushroom Braised Pot Roast

Preparation Time: 10 minutes

Cooking Time: 1 hour 30 minutes

Servings: 10

Ingredients:

- 4 pounds chuck roast
- 2 tablespoons vegetable oil
- 1/2 teaspoon salt
- 1/4 teaspoon pepper
- 1 cup chopped onion
- 2 cups beef broth
- 2 tablespoons gravy master
- 2 tablespoons butter
- 1-pound cremini mushrooms sliced or white button mushrooms
- 1/2 teaspoon salt

Directions:

Season roast with salt and pepper. Add vegetable oil to the Instant Pot. Sear roast on all sides until brown. Add 1 chopped onion to the Instant Pot along with 2 cups of beef broth, and 2 tablespoons of

Gravy Master. Use the meat-setting button for 90 minutes. Allow the pot to release by using the natural release method. While the pot is releasing the pressure, naturally sauté 1 pound of sliced mushrooms butter. Add 1/2 teaspoon of salt to the mushrooms while sautéing. When mushrooms are cooked through, add to the roast.

Nutrition:
Calories: 392, Carbohydrates: 3g, Protein: 37g, Fat: 26g, Saturated Fat: 12g, Sugar: 1g, Cholesterol: 131mg, Sodium: 782mg, Fiber: 0g, Potassium: 862mg

20. Shepherd's Pie

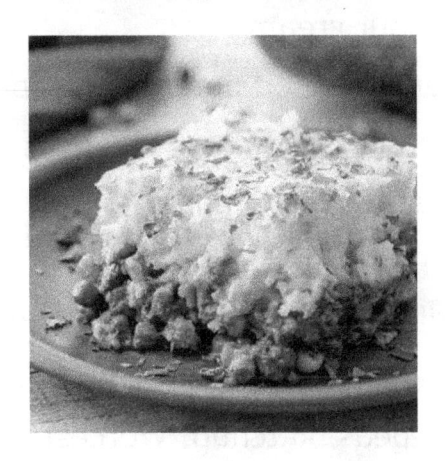

Preparation time: 10 minutes

Cooking time: 20 minutes

Servings: 4

Ingredients:

- 1-pound ground beef
- 1 cup onion, diced
- 2 cups frozen corn, thawed
- 2 cups frozen peas, thawed
- 2 tablespoons ketchup
- 1 tablespoon Worcestershire sauce
- 2 teaspoons garlic, minced
- 1 tablespoon cornstarch
- 1 teaspoon beef bouillon granules

- ½ cup cold water
- ½ cup sour cream
- 3 ½ cups mashed potatoes (prepared with milk and butter)
- ¾ cup shredded cheddar cheese

Directions:

In a large skillet, brown the ground beef and onion over medium-high heat. Drain off any excess fat. Add the corn, peas, ketchup, Worcestershire sauce, and garlic. Stir well to combine, and then reduce the heat to medium low and cook for approximately 5 minutes, or until mixture the becomes bubbly. Make a slurry by stirring the corn starch and bouillon into the ½ cup of water. Stir until it is smooth, then stir it into the beef mixture and cook for about 2 more minutes. Stir in the sour cream and heat through. Cover the mixture with the mashed potatoes, and sprinkle on the cheese. Place the lid on the skillet and cook until the cheese melts. Serve.

Nutrition:

Calories: 693, Total Fat: 40g, Saturated Fat: 17g, Cholesterol: 174mg, Sodium: 1481mg, Potassium: 1499mg, Carbohydrates: 52g

21. Steak Diane

Preparation time: 10 minutes

Cooking time: 15 minutes

Servings: 2

Ingredients:

- 2–3 tablespoons butter
- 12 ounces beef tenderloin, cut into
- 3-ounce medallions Salt to taste
- 2 teaspoons cracked whole black peppercorns
- ½ cup fresh mushrooms, sliced
- 3 tablespoons pearl onions, chopped
- ¼ cup brandy or white wine
- 1 teaspoon Worcestershire sauce
- 1 tablespoon Dijon mustard
- ¾ cup beef stock
- ¼ cup cream

Directions:

Preheat the oven to 350°F. In a large skillet, melt 2 tablespoons of the butter over medium-high heat. Sprinkle both sides of the beef medallions with salt and fresh pepper. Sear them for about 2 minutes on each side, and then remove them from the skillet to an ovenproof dish and transfer it to the oven to keep warm. While those are in the oven, add a bit more butter to the skillet. Add the mushrooms and pearl onions and cook until they start to turn soft. Add the white wine and Worcestershire, then stir in the mustard. Cook for about 2 minutes. Stir in the beef stock and bring it to a boil. When it boils, remove it from the heat and stir in the cream. Remove the beef from the oven and plate it with sauce over the top.

Nutrition:
Calories: 328.7, Total Fat: 21.7 g, Protein: 22.5g, Cholesterol: 78.9mg, Sodium: 312.5 mg, Sugars: 1.1g, Potassium: 403.9mg, Carbohydrate: 4.5g,

22. Grilled Steak Medallions

Preparation time: 10 minutes
Cooking time: 35 minutes
Servings: 8

Ingredients:

- 1-pound sirloin steak, cut into medallions or individual pieces
- Salt and pepper to taste
- 1 tablespoon extra-virgin olive oil
- 3 tablespoons unsalted butter
- 3 cups mushrooms, sliced
- 1 medium-large shallot, minced
- 1 tablespoon garlic, minced
- 10 asparagus spears, chopped at an angle
- 1 cup grape tomatoes, halved
- 2 tablespoons flour
- ½ cup red wine
- ½ cup low-sodium beef broth
- ¼ teaspoon dried thyme, or one sprig of fresh thyme 1 bay leaf

Directions:

Season the meat with salt and pepper. In a large skillet, heat the olive oil until it is hot. Add the steaks and cook for 4 minutes on the first side without moving them. After 4 minutes, flip and cook an additional 2 minutes. Remove the steaks from the skillet and cover with foil to keep them warm. Add 3 tablespoons of butter to the skillet. After it melts, add the mushrooms, shallots, garlic, and asparagus. Let them cook for 2-3 minutes, then stir and continue cooking until the asparagus starts to get soft. Add the grape tomatoes to heat them through. Add the flour and stir to combine, and then whisk in the red wine, beef broth, thyme, and bay leaf. Bring to a boil and cook until it starts to thicken. Remove the bay leaf before serving. Serve steak medallions with sauce and vegetables on top.

Nutrition:

Calories: 440, Total Fat: 19g, Sugars: 6g Cholesterol: 140mg, Sodium: 1320mg, Carbohydrates: 24g, Dietary Fiber: 4g, Protein: 45g

23. Provolone Stuffed Meatballs

Preparation time: 15 minutes
Cooking time: 25 minutes
Servings: 4

Ingredients:

- ½ pound ground beef
- ½ pound ground veal
- 1-pound ground pork
- ½ cup breadcrumbs
- 2 tablespoons fresh parsley (minced)
- 1 egg (slightly beaten)
- ⅓ cup milk
- 3 cloves garlic, minced
- 1 teaspoon salt
- ½ teaspoon ground black pepper
- 3 ounces provolone cheese, cut into cubes
- 2 tablespoons olive oil
- 2 cups marinara sauce
- 2 cups alfredo sauce
- 1-pound fettuccine pasta
- ¼ cup chopped fresh parsley for serving

- ½ cup Parmesan cheese, grated, for serving

Directions:

In a large bowl, mix together the beef, veal, pork, breadcrumbs, parsley, egg, milk, garlic, salt, and pepper. Mix with your hands to make sure it is completely blended. Form into meatballs, but do not overwork the meat or your meatballs will be tough. Press your thumb into the balls as you form them and place a cube of the cheese inside. Reform the meatball around it.

In a heavy skillet, heat 2 teaspoons of olive oil over medium-high heat. When the oil is hot, add the meatballs, and brown them on all sides. When they are browned, transfer the balls to a plate line with paper towels to drain. (They will finish cooking in the sauce.) Transfer the meatballs to a medium-sized saucepan and add the marinara sauce. Cook over medium to low heat for about 25 minutes. Cook your fettuccine in a pot of boiling water until al dente, drain, and return to the pot. Add the Alfredo sauce. Heat and stir until the Alfredo sauce is hot. To serve, place a bed of the fettuccine with Alfredo sauce on a serving plate, and scoop on some meatballs with a bit of marinara over the top. Sprinkle with fresh parsley and Parmesan.

Nutrition:
Calories: 1550, Total Fat: 97g, Saturated Fat: 46g,
Trans Fat: 2.5g,   Sugars: 0g,   Cholesterol 0mg,
Sodium: 3910mg,   Protein: 58g,
Total Carbohydrates: 113g,   Dietary Fiber: 9g,

24. Brunch Burger

Preparation time: 10 minutes

Cooking time: 30 minutes

Servings: 2

Ingredients:

- 4 thick-cut bacon slices
- ½ pound ground beef
- Salt and pepper to taste
- 2–4 slices cheddar cheese
- 1 russet potato
- ½ small onion
- 3 eggs
- 2 tablespoons flour
- 2 tablespoons vegetable oil
- 2 sesame hamburger buns

Directions:

Cook the bacon in a skillet until crisp. When it is done, remove it from the skillet and set it on a plate lined with paper towel to drain. Season the ground beef with salt and pepper and form it into loose patties.

Cook the burgers in the bacon grease on medium-high heat until they reach your desired doneness. Just before they are done cooking, top with a portion of the cheese. Cover, and set aside. Peel the potato and grate it into a small bowl. Grate the onion in as well. Add 1 egg, salt, pepper, and flour. Heat a clean skillet over medium-high heat and add the oil. Form the potato mixture into 2 potato pancakes and transfer them to the skillet, cooking on each side for about 3-4 minutes, or until crisp. Transfer them to a paper towel lined plate to drain. Break the remaining eggs into the skillet and cook for about 3 minutes according to your preference. Assemble your burger on a bun with bacon, egg, a potato pancake, and whatever other toppings you enjoy.

Nutrition:

Calories: 1240, Total Fat: 80 g, Cholesterol: 360mg, Sodium: 2380 mg, Protein:65g, Sugars:13g, Total Carbohydrate:64g, Dietary Fiber: 5

25. Quesadilla Burger

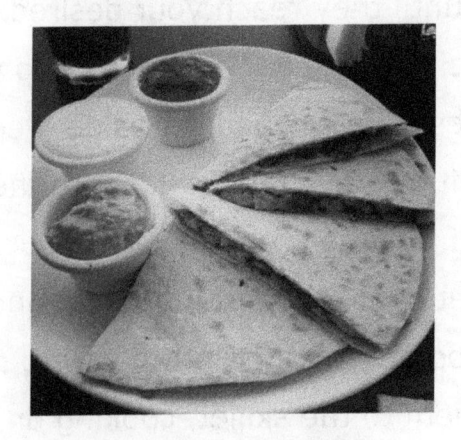

Preparation time: 15 minutes

Cooking time: 15 minutes

Servings: 4

Ingredients:

- 1 ½ pounds ground beef
- 8 (6-inch) flour tortillas
- 1 tablespoon butter

Tex-Mex seasoning for the burgers:

- 2 teaspoons ground cumin
- 2 tablespoons paprika
- 1 teaspoon black pepper
- ½ teaspoon cayenne pepper, more or less depending on taste

- 1 teaspoon salt or to taste
- 1 tablespoon dried oregano

Toppings:
- 8 slices pepper jack cheese
- 4 slices Applewood-smoked bacon, cooked and crumbled
- ½ cup shredded iceberg lettuce

Pico de Galo:
- 1-2 Roma tomatoes, deseeded and diced thin
- ½-1 tablespoon thinly diced onion (red or yellow is fine)
- 1-2 teaspoons fresh lime juice
- 1-2 teaspoons fresh cilantro, chopped finely
- 1-2 teaspoons thinly diced jalapeños pepper
- Salt and pepper to taste

Tex-Mex ranch dressing:
- ½ cup sour cream
- ½ cup ranch dressing such as Hidden Valley
- 1 teaspoon Tex-Mex seasoning
- ¼ cup mild salsa
- Pepper to taste

For serving (optional):
- Guacamole, and sour cream

Directions:

In a mixing bowl, combine the Tex-Mex seasoning ingredients and stir to ensure they are well combined. Prepare the fresh Pico de Gallo by mixing all the ingredients in a bowl. Set aside in the refrigerator until ready to use. Prepare the Tex-Mex ranch dressing by mixing all the ingredients in a bowl. Set aside in the refrigerator until ready to use. Add 2 tablespoons of the Tex-Mex seasoning to the ground beef and mix it in, being careful not to overwork the beef or your burgers will be tough. Form into 4 large ¼-inch thick burger patties and cook either on the grill or in a skillet to your preference. Heat a clean skillet over medium-low heat. Butter each of the flour tortillas on one side. Place one butter side down in the skillet. Top with 1 slice of cheese, some shredded lettuce, some Pico de Gallo, some bacon, and then top with a cooked burger. Top the burger with some of the Tex-Mex ranch dressing sauce to taste, some Pico the Gallo, bacon, and another slice of cheese. Cover with another tortilla, butter side up. Cook for about 1 minute or until the tortilla is golden. Then carefully flip the tortilla and cook until the cheese has melted. This step can be done in a sandwich press if you have one. Cut the tortillas in quarters or halves and serve with a side of the Tex-Mex ranch dressing, guacamole, and sour cream, if desired.

Nutrition:

Calories: 1330, Total Fat: 93 g, Sugars: 7 g, Cholesterol: 240mg, Sodium: 3000mg, Total Carbohydrate: 50g, Dietary Fiber: 6g, Protein: 74 g

26. Honey Barbecue Riblets

Preparation time: 25 minutes

Cooking time: 2-5 hours

Servings: 4

Ingredients:

- 2 racks pork baby back ribs (or riblets if you can find them), about 2 ¼ pounds
- Salt to taste
- Pepper to taste
- Garlic powder to taste
- ½ teaspoon liquid smoke

For the sauce:

- 1 cup ketchup
- ½ cup corn syrup
- ½ cup honey
- ¼ cup apple cider vinegar
- ¼ cup water
- 2 tablespoons molasses
- 2 teaspoons dry mustard
- 2 teaspoons garlic powder
- 1 teaspoon chili powder

- 1 teaspoon onion powder
- ¼ teaspoon liquid smoke flavor

Directions:

Preheat the oven to 275°F. Season the ribs with salt, pepper, and garlic powder. Place a wire rack in the bottom of a large roasting pan. Pour in about a half a cup of water and ½ teaspoon of liquid smoke. Place the ribs on the rack, making sure they are not touching the liquid. Seal the roasting pan with either the lid or aluminum foil. Place the pan in the oven and cook for 2–5 hours, depending on how many ribs you are cooking. Check every so often for desired tenderness. (You can speed this process up if you have an Instant Pot or other pressure cooker.) Meanwhile, in a medium saucepan, combine all the ingredients for the sauce and bring it to a boil. Reduce the heat and let it simmer for 20 minutes. When the ribs have reached the desired tenderness, remove them from the oven and place them on a baking sheet. Set the oven to broil. Brush the ribs with barbecue sauce and broil until the sauce starts to turn a little brown/black. Be careful not to let it burn. Remove the ribs from the oven and serve with additional barbecue sauce.

Nutrition:

Calories: 693.4, Total Fat: 44.8 g, Protein: 37.0, Cholesterol: 178.6 mg, Sodium: 804.2 mg, Potassium: 500.3 mg, g, Sugars: 34.1 g, Total Carbohydrate: 35.5 g, Dietary Fiber: 0.2g,

27. Cilantro Beef Curry

Preparation time: 10 minutes
Cooking time: 30 minutes

Servings: 4

Ingredients:

- 2 pounds beef stew meat, cubed
- ¼ cup cilantro, chopped
- 1 yellow onion, chopped
- 3 garlic cloves, minced
- ½ cup tomatoes, crushed
- Salt and black pepper to the taste
- 1 tablespoon garam masala
- 1 teaspoon turmeric powder
- ½ teaspoon coriander, ground
- ½ teaspoon cumin, ground
- ½ teaspoon cayenne pepper
- 1 teaspoon brown sugar
- 1 tablespoon vegetable oil
- ½ teaspoon lemon zest, grated
- 1 cup beef stock

Directions:

Set the instant pot on Sauté mode, add the oil, heat it up, add the meat, onion, garlic, masala, turmeric and coriander, stir and brown for 10 minutes. Add the rest of the Ingredients, toss, put the lid on and cook on High for 20 minutes. Release the pressure naturally for 10 minutes; divide the mix into bowls and Serve.

Nutrition:

Calories: 481, Fat: 17.9, Fiber: 1.2, Carbs: 5.7, Protein: 70.3

28. Coconut Ribs Curry

Preparation time: 10 minutes

Cooking time: 35 minutes

Servings: 4

Ingredients:

- 2 pounds beef ribs
- 1 yellow onion, chopped
- 1 teaspoon garam masala
- 2 tablespoons tomato paste
- 4 garlic cloves, minced
- 1 tablespoon red curry paste
- 14 ounces coconut cream
- 3 cups beef stock
- ½ cup basil, chopped
- 1 tablespoon fish sauce
- 1 pound cauliflower florets
- 2 bay leaves
- 1 tablespoon sunflower oil
- Salt and black pepper to the taste

Directions:

Set the instant pot on Sauté mode, add the oil, heat it up, add the ribs, onion, garlic, curry paste, and the garam masala, stir and brown for 5 minutes. Add the remaining Ingredients, put the lid don and cook on High for 30 minutes. Release the pressure naturally for 10 minutes; divide everything into bowls and Serve.

Nutrition:

Calories: 76, Fat: 42, Fiber: 6.1, Protein: 17.6

29. Creamy Coconut Pork

Preparation time: 10 minutes

Cooking time: 30 minutes

Servings: 6

Ingredients:

- 2 cups beef stock
- 2 pounds pork stew meat, cubed
- 4 garlic cloves, minced
- 1 leek, sliced
- ½ cup coconut, shredded
- 1 teaspoon garam masala
- ½ teaspoon cumin, ground
- 1 teaspoon sage, dried
- ½ cup heavy cream
- 1 tablespoon coconut oil
- Salt and black pepper to the taste

Directions:

Set the instant pot on Sauté mode, add the oil, heat it up, and add the meat, garlic and the leek and brown for 5 minutes. Add the rest of the Ingredients, toss, put the lid on and cook on High for 25 minutes.

Release the pressure naturally for 10 minutes; divide everything into bowls and Serve.

Nutrition:
Calories: 377, Fat: 15.7, Fiber: 6.7, Carbs: 22.3, Protein: 14.3

30. Madras Tomato Beef

Preparation time: 10 minutes
Cooking time: 30 minutes
Servings: 4

Ingredients:

- 1 tablespoon cumin, ground
- 2 tablespoons coriander, ground
- 1 teaspoon turmeric powder
- 1 teaspoon chili powder
- Salt and black pepper to the taste
- 2 teaspoons ginger, grated
- 2 garlic cloves, minced
- 2 tablespoons lemon juice
- 2 pounds beef stew meat, cubed
- 2 tablespoons canola oil
- 1 cup beef stock
- 2 tablespoons tomato paste
- 1 tablespoon mint, chopped

Directions:

Set the instant pot on Sauté mode, add the oil, heat it up, add the meat, garlic, ginger, chili powder, turmeric, coriander and the cumin, stir and brown for 5 minutes. Add the rest of the Ingredients, put the lid on and cook on High for 25 minutes. Release the pressure naturally for 10 minutes; divide the mix into bowls and Serve.

Nutrition:

Calories 399, Fat 16.6, Fiber 7.7, Carbs: 26.5, Protein 12.7

31. Ginger Beef Curry

Preparation time: 10 minutes
Cooking time: 35 minutes
Servings: 4

Ingredients:

- 2 tablespoons vegetable oil
- 1 yellow onion, chopped
- 12 curry leaves, chopped
- 6 garlic cloves, minced
- 4 teaspoons ginger, grated
- 1 tablespoon tomato paste
- 2 teaspoons coriander, ground
- 1 cup water
- 1 teaspoon garam masala
- ½ teaspoon turmeric powder
- 4 star anise
- Salt and black pepper to the taste
- 2 pounds beef short ribs, cut into medium pieces

Directions:

Set the instant pot on Sauté mode, add the oil, heat it up, add the onion, garlic, curry leaves, ginger and the meat and brown for 5 minutes. Add the rest of the Ingredients, toss, put the lid on and cook on High for 30 minutes. Release the pressure naturally for 10 minutes; divide the mix into bowls and Serve.

Nutrition:

Calories: 353, Fat: 14.4, Fiber: 4.5, Carbs: 22.3, Protein: 46

32. Beef with Cardamom Veggies

Preparation time: 10 minutes
Cooking time: 25 minutes

Servings: 6

Ingredients:

- 2 pound beef stew meat, cut into strips
- 2 yellow onions, chopped
- 2 tomatoes, cubed
- 2 tablespoons ginger paste
- 2 tablespoons garlic paste
- 3 green chilies, chopped
- 2 tablespoons coriander seeds
- 4 tablespoons fennel seeds
- 8 cloves
- 6 cardamom pods
- 1 tablespoon black peppercorns, crushed
- 10 curry leaves, chopped
- 1 cup coconut, shredded
- 1 tablespoon mustard seeds
- 2 tablespoons sunflower oil

Directions:

Set the instant pot on Sauté mode, add the oil, heat it up, add the meat, onions, garlic and ginger paste, stir and brown for 5 minutes. Add the rest of the Ingredients, put the lid on and cook on High for 20 minutes.

Release the pressure naturally for 10 minutes; divide the mix into bowls and Serve.

Nutrition:

Calories: 344, Fat: 12.4, Fiber: 6.6, Carbs: 19.9, Protein: 25

33. Onion Beef in Yogurt

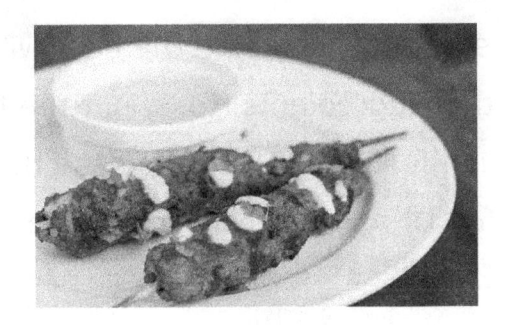

Preparation time: 10 minutes
Cooking time: 30 minutes
Servings: 4

Ingredients:

- 1 pound beef stew meat, cubed
- 4 garlic cloves, minced
- 2 cups yellow onion, chopped
- 1 tablespoon ginger, grated
- 1 cup yogurt
- 2 bay leaves
- 1 teaspoon sweet paprika
- 2 tablespoons curry powder
- 1 teaspoon garam masala
- 2 tablespoons lemon juice

- Salt and black pepper to the taste

Directions:

In your instant pot, combine the beef with the garlic and the other Ingredients, toss, put the lid on and cook on High for 30 minutes. Release the pressure naturally for 10 minutes; divide the mix into bowls and Serve.

Nutrition:

Calories: 388, Fat: 15.5, Fiber: 5.67, Carbs: 25.5, Protein: 22

34. Ginger Beef Mix

Preparation time: 10 minutes
Cooking time: 30 minutes
Servings: 4

Ingredients:

- 2 pounds beef stew meat, cubed
- 1 tablespoon garlic, minced
- 1-inch ginger, grated
- 2 cups red onion, chopped
- 2 tablespoons lemon juice
- 2 teaspoons coriander powder
- 2 teaspoons meat masala
- 2 teaspoons chili powder
- 1 teaspoon turmeric powder
- ½ cup water
- Salt to the taste

Directions:

In your instant pot, combine the meat with the garlic, ginger and the other Ingredients, toss, put the lid on and cook on High for 30 minutes. Release the pressure naturally for 10 minutes; divide everything into bowls and Serve.

Nutrition:

Calories: 388, Fat: 14.5, Fiber: 5.5,
Carbs: 22, Protein: 17

35. Beef and Lentils Curry

Preparation time: 10 minutes
Cooking time: 35 minutes
Servings: 4

Ingredients:

- ¼ cup vegetable oil
- 1 tablespoon coriander, ground
- 1 teaspoon cumin seeds
- 1 yellow onion, chopped
- 4 garlic cloves, minced
- 1 tablespoon ginger, grated
- 2 pounds beef stew meat, cubed
- 14 ounces canned tomatoes, chopped
- 1 teaspoon turmeric powder
- 2 cups water
- ½ cup green lentils, rinsed
- 1 green chili, chopped
- Salt and black pepper to the taste

Directions:

Set the instant pot on Sauté mode, add the oil, heat it up, add the meat, ginger, garlic and onion, stir and brown for 5 minutes. Add the coriander, cumin and the other Ingredients, toss, put the lid on and cook on High for 30 minutes. Release the pressure naturally for 10 minutes; divide the mix into bowls and Serve.

Nutrition:

Calories: 372, Fat: 15.5, Fiber: 6.6, Carbs: 19.8, Protein 22

36. Curry Pork with Lentils

Preparation time: 10 minutes
Cooking time: 30 minutes
Servings: 4

Ingredients:

- 1 pound pork stew meat, cubed
- ½ cup curry paste
- 2 teaspoons vegetable oil
- 2 garlic cloves, minced
- 1 yellow onion, chopped
- 1 cup red lentils
- 2 teaspoons ginger, grated
- 1 and ½ cups beef stock
- 1 cup coconut milk
- 2 tablespoons coriander, chopped

Directions:

Set the instant pot on Sauté mode, add the oil, heat it up, add the meat, onion and the garlic and sauté for 5 minutes. Add the rest of the Ingredients, put the lid on and cook on High for 25 minutes. Release the pressure naturally for 10 minutes; divide the mix into bowls and Serve.

Nutrition:

Calories: 356, Fat: 16.5, Fiber: 4.5, Carbs: 22, Protein: 4.65

37. Ground Beef Masala

Preparation time: 10 minutes
Cooking time: 20 minutes
Servings: 4

Ingredients:

- 2 pounds beef, ground
- 1 red onion, chopped
- 10 garlic cloves, minced
- 2 tablespoons cumin powder
- 2 green chilies, chopped
- 1 tablespoon coriander, ground
- 1 tomato, cubed
- ½ cup dill, chopped
- 1 potato, peeled and cubed
- Salt and black pepper to the taste
- ¼ cup beef stock

Directions:

In your instant pot, combine the beef with the onion, garlic and the other Ingredients, toss, put the lid on and cook on High for 20 minutes. Release the pressure naturally for 10 minutes, divide the mix between plates and serve...

Nutrition:

Calories: 254, Fat: 12, Fiber: 2,
Carbs: 14.6, Protein: 16

38. Chili Beef and Peas

Preparation time: 10 minutes
Cooking time: 20 minutes
Servings: 4

Ingredients:

- 1-inch ginger, grated
- 2 pounds beef meat, ground
- 2 tablespoons canola oil
- 2 garlic cloves, minced
- 1 chili pepper, minced
- 1 teaspoon garam masala
- 2 tomatoes, cubed
- Salt and black pepper to the taste
- ½ cup peas
- ¼ cup cilantro, chopped
- ¼ cup beef stock

Directions:

Set the instant pot on Sauté mode, add the oil, heat it up, and add the garlic, chili pepper and the meat and brown for 5 minutes. Add the rest of the Ingredients, toss, put the lid on and cook on High for

15 minutes. Release the pressure naturally for 10 minutes; divide the mix between plates and Serve.

Nutrition:

Calories: 343, Fat: 15, Fiber: 3,
Carbs: 14.6, Protein: 20

39. Coconut Masala Beef

Preparation time: 10 minutes
Cooking time: 25 minutes
Servings: 4

Ingredients:

- 2 tablespoons canola oil
- 2 pounds beef stew meat, cubed
- 1 teaspoon garam masala
- ½ teaspoon coriander, ground
- 2 and ½ tablespoons curry powder
- 2 yellow onions, chopped
- Salt and black pepper to the taste
- 2 garlic cloves, minced
- 10 ounces coconut milk
- 2 tablespoons cilantro, chopped

Directions:

Set your instant pot on Sauté mode, add the oil, heat it up, and add the meat, garam masala, coriander, onions and garlic and brown for 5 minutes. Add the rest of the Ingredients, put the lid on and cook on High for 20 minutes. Release the pressure naturally for 10 minutes; divide everything between plates and Serve.

Nutrition:

Calories: 363g, Fat: 16g, Fiber: 3, Carbs: 15.6g, Protein: 1g

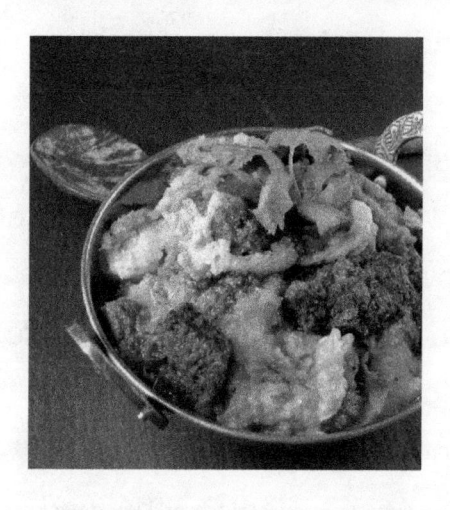

40. Grilled Steak Salad with Blue Cheese Dressing

Preparation time: 5 Minutes

Cooking time: 16 Minutes

Servings: 4 to 6

Ingredients:

- 4 (8-ounce) skirt steaks
- Sea salt
- Freshly ground black pepper
- 6 cups chopped romaine lettuce
- ¾ cup cherry tomatoes, halved
- ¼ cup blue cheese, crumbled
- 1 cup croutons
- 2 avocados, peeled and sliced
- 1 cup blue cheese dressing

Directions:

Insert the Grill Grate and close the hood. Select GRILL, set the temperature to HIGH, and set the time to 8 minutes. Select START/STOP to begin preheating. Season the steaks on both sides with the salt and pepper. When the unit beeps to signify it has preheated, place 2 steaks on the Grill Grate. Gently press the steaks down to maximize grill marks. Close the hood and cook for 4 minutes. After 4 minutes, flip the steaks, close the hood, and cook for an additional 4 minutes. Remove the steaks from the grill and transfer to them a cutting board. Tent with aluminum foil.Repeat step 3 with the remaining 2 steaks. While the second set of steaks is cooking, assemble the salad by tossing together the lettuce, tomatoes, blue cheese crumbles, and croutons. Top with the avocado slices.

Once the second set of steaks has finished cooking, slice all four of the steaks into thin strips, and place on top of the salad. Drizzle with the blue cheese dressing and Serve.

Nutrition:

Calories: 911,   Total fat: 67g, Sodium: 1062mg, Saturated fat: 18g,   Cholesterol: 167mg

41. Filet Mignon with Pineapple Salsa

Preparation time: 15 minutes
Cooking time: 8 minutes
Servings: 4

Ingredients:

- Sea salt
- 4 (6- to 8-ounce) filet mignon steaks
- 1 tablespoon canola oil, divided
- Freshly ground black pepper
- ½ medium pineapple, cored and diced
- 1 medium red onion, diced
- 1 jalapeño pepper, seeded, stemmed, and diced
- 1 tablespoon freshly squeezed lime juice
- ¼ cup chopped fresh cilantro leaves
- Chili powder
- Ground coriander

Directions:

Rub each filet on all sides with ½ tablespoon of the oil, then season with the salt and pepper. Insert the

Grill Grate and close the hood. Select GRILL, set temperature to HIGH, and set time to 8 minutes. Select START/STOP to begin preheating. When the unit beeps to signify it has preheated, add the filets to the Grill Grate. Gently press the filets down to maximize grill marks, and then close the hood. After 4 minutes, open the hood and flip the filets. Close the hood and continue cooking for an additional 4 minutes or until the filets' internal temperature reads 125°F on a food thermometer. Remove the filets from the grill; they will continue to cook (called carry-over cooking) to a food-safe temperature even after you've removed them from the grill. Let the filets rest for a total of 10 minutes; this allows the natural juices to redistribute into the steak. While the filets rest, in a medium bowl, combine the pineapple, onion, and jalapeño. Stir in the lime juice and cilantro, then season to taste with the chili powder and coriander. Plate the filets, and pile the salsa on top of each before serving.

VARIATION TIP: There are so many ways to put your own twist on this recipe. Try using other cuts of beef, like flank steak or New York strip, or different salsa variations depending on the season, like fresh mango, Pico de Gallo, or salsa Verde.

Nutrition:
Calories: 571;   Total fat: 25g;   Sodium: 264mg
Saturated fat: 8g;   Cholesterol: 192mg;

42. Chili-Rubbed Flank Steak

Preparation time: 10 Minutes
Cooking time: 8 Minutes
Servings: 2

Ingredients:

- 1 tablespoon chili powder
- 1 teaspoon dried oregano
- 2 teaspoons ground cumin
- 1 teaspoon sea salt
- ¼ teaspoon freshly ground black pepper
- 2 (8-ounce) flank steaks

Directions:

Insert the Grill Grate and close the hood. Select GRILL, set the temperature to HIGH, and set the time to 8 minutes. Select START/STOP to begin preheating. In a small bowl, mix together the chili powder, oregano, cumin, salt, and pepper. Use your hands to rub the spice mixture on all sides of the steaks. When the unit beeps to signify it has preheated, place the steaks on the Grill Grate. Gently press the steaks down to maximize grill marks. Close the hood and cook for 4 minutes. After 4 minutes, flip the steaks, close the hood, and cook for 4 minutes more. Remove the steaks from the grill, and transfer them to a cutting board. Let rest for 5 minutes before slicing and serve.

Nutrition:

Calories: 363;   Total fat: 15g;   Sodium: 1008mg, Saturated fat: 6g;   Cholesterol: 100mg;

43. Soy and Garlic Steak Kebabs

Preparation time: 5 minutes, plus 30 minutes to marinate

Cooking time: 12 minutes

Servings: 4

Ingredients:

- ¾ cup soy sauce
- 5 garlic cloves, minced
- 3 tablespoons sesame oil
- ½ cup canola oil
- ⅓ cup sugar
- ¼ teaspoon dried ground ginger
- 2 (10- to 12-ounce) New York strip steaks, cut in 2-inch cubes
- 1 cup whole white mushrooms
- 1 red bell pepper, seeded, and cut into 2 inch cubes
- 1 red onion, cut into 2-inch wedges

Directions:

In a medium bowl, whisk together the soy sauce, garlic, sesame oil, canola oil, sugar, and ginger until well combined. Add the steak and toss to coat. Cover and refrigerate for at least 30 minutes. Insert the Grill Grate and close the hood. Select GRILL, set the temperature to MEDIUM, and set the time to 12 minutes. Select START/STOP to begin preheating. While the unit is preheating, assemble the skewers in the following order: steak, mushroom, bell pepper, onion. Ensure the Ingredients are pushed almost completely down to the end of the skewers. When the unit beeps to signify it has preheated, place the skewers on the Grill Grate. Close the hood and cook for 8 minutes without flipping. After 8 minutes, check the steak for desired doneness, cooking up to 4 minutes more if desired. When cooking is complete, Serve immediately.

SUBSTITUTION TIP: While you can swap the steak for chicken or shrimp, I recommend sticking with New York strip or top sirloin. These cuts have great flavor and are very tender when marinated and grilled.

Nutrition:

Calories: 647, Total fat: 45g, Sodium: 1001mg, Saturated fat: 12g, Cholesterol: 135mg

44. Beef Bulgogi

Preparation time: 5 minutes, plus 1 hour to marinate

Cooking time: 5 minutes

Servings: 4

Ingredients:

- ⅓ cup soy sauce
- 2 tablespoons sesame oil
- 2½ tablespoons brown sugar
- 3 garlic cloves, minced
- ½ teaspoon freshly ground black pepper
- 1 pound rib eye steak, thinly sliced
- 2 scallions, thinly sliced, for garnish
- Toasted sesame seeds, for garnish

Directions:

In a small bowl, whisk together the soy sauce, sesame oil, brown sugar, garlic, and black pepper until fully combined. Place the beef into a large shallow bowl, and pour the sauce over the slices. Cover and refrigerate for 1 hour. Insert the Grill Grate and close the hood. Select GRILL, set the temperature to MEDIUM, and set the time to 5 minutes. Select START/STOP to begin preheating. When the unit beeps to signify it has preheated, place the beef onto the Grill Grate. Close the hood and cook for 4 minutes without flipping. After 4 minutes, check the steak for desired doneness, cooking for up to 1 minute more, if desired. When cooking is complete, top with scallions and sesame seeds and Serve immediately.

HACK IT: To make the steak easier to slice, stick it in the freezer for an hour before you cut it and put it in the marinade.

Nutrition:
Calories: 403; Cholesterol: 76mg; Sodium: 1263mg
Total fat: 31g; Saturated fat: 13g;

45. Gochujang-Marinated Baby Back Ribs

Preparation time: 10 Minutes, Plus 6 Hours to Marinate

Cooking time: 22 Minutes

Servings: 4

Ingredients:

- ¼ cup gochujang paste
- ¼ cup soy sauce
- ¼ cup freshly squeezed orange juice
- 2 tablespoons apple cider vinegar
- 2 tablespoons sesame oil
- 6 garlic cloves, minced
- 1½ tablespoons brown sugar
- 1 tablespoon grated fresh ginger
- 1 teaspoon salt
- 4 (8- to 10-ounce) baby back ribs

Directions:

In a medium bowl, add the gochujang paste, soy sauce, orange juice, vinegar, oil, garlic, sugar, ginger, and salt, and stir to combine. Place the baby back ribs on a baking sheet and coat all sides with the sauce. Cover with aluminum foil and refrigerate for 6 hours. Insert the Grill Grate and close the hood. Select GRILL, set the temperature to MEDIUM, and set the time to 22 minutes. Select START/STOP to begin preheating. When the unit beeps to signify it has preheated, place the ribs on the Grill Grate. Close the hood and cook for 11 minutes. After 11 minutes, flip the ribs, close the hood, and cook for an additional 11 minutes. When cooking is complete, serve immediately.

SUBSTITUTION TIP: Don't have orange juice? Try swapping in another citrusy juice here, like lime or lemon.

Nutrition:
Calories: 826; Cholesterol: 191mg;
Sodium: 2113mg, Total fat: 64g;
Saturated fat: 22g;

46. Chili's Boneless Buffalo Wings

Preparation time: 30 minutes

Cooking time: 15 minutes

Servings: 2

Ingredients:
- 1 cup flour
- 2 teaspoons salt
- ½ teaspoon black pepper, ground
- ¼ teaspoon cayenne pepper, ground
- 1 egg
- 1 cup milk
- 5 cups vegetable oil
- 2 chicken breasts, boneless and skinless, cut into 6 pieces
- ¼ cup hot sauce
- 1 tablespoon margarine
- 1 blue cheese salad dressing
- 1 stalk celery, cut into sticks

Directions:

In a bowl, mix together flour, salt, peppers, and paprika. Add egg and milk to a separate bowl and mix well. Preheat 5 cups oil in a deep-fryer to 375 °F. Coat chicken pieces into egg mixture. Allow excess to drip off, then coat with flour mixture. Repeat twice for a double coat. Transfer breaded chicken onto a plate and refrigerate for about 15 minutes. Deep-fry each for about 5 minutes or until brown and transfer onto a paper towel-lined plate. Meanwhile, mix hot sauce and margarine in a bowl. Then, heat in the microwave for about 20 seconds or until melted. Mix well until fully blended. Place chicken pieces in a large Ziplock bag and add sauce. Seal bag tightly. Using your hands, mix chicken and sauce together until well-coated.

Serve chicken pieces on a plate with blue cheese dressing and celery sticks on the side.

Nutrition:

Calories: 398, Fat: 13 g, Carbs: 55 g, Protein: 14 g

47. Crunchy Pork Wontons

Preparation time: 10 minutes

Cooking time: 15 minutes

Servings: 3

Ingredients:

- ¾ pound ground pork
- 6 wonton wrappers
- 1 tablespoon olive oil
- 3 tablespoons onion, finely chopped
- 1 habanero pepper, minced
- 1 red bell pepper, deseeded and chopped
- 1 green bell pepper, deseeded and chopped
- Salt and ground black pepper, to taste
- 1 teaspoon dried thyme
- ½ teaspoon dried parsley flakes
- Cooking spray

Directions:

To make the filling, in a skillet, warm the olive oil over medium heat. Add the ground pork, onions, habanero pepper, bell peppers, salt, and black pepper. Cook them until soft and aromatic, around 4 minutes. Put in the thyme and parsley flakes and mix well. Transfer the mixture in the skillet to a bowl. Allow it to cool. To make wontons, dust your hand with a touch of flour. Unfold a wonton wrapper in your palm and scoop ½ tablespoon of the filling in the center. Seal the wonton by pressing the wrapper's edges together with your fingers. Repeat with the remaining wrappers. Spritz the air fryer basket with cooking spray. Arrange the prepared wontons in the basket. Put the air fryer lid on and cook in batches in the preheated instant pot at 350ºF for 12 minutes. Remove from the basket and Serve warm with vinegar, if desired.

Nutrition:

Calories: 295, Fat: 14.4g, Carbs: 21.7g, Protein: 18.2g, Sugars: 1.6g

48. Buffalo Chicken & Blue Cheese Slaw

Preparation Time: 30 mins

Cooking Time: 1 hr

Serves: 4

Ingredients:

- 8 skin-on, bone-in chicken thighs
- 100ml hot sauce
- 2tsp smoked paprika
- 1tbsp light brown soft sugar
- 1tbsp white wine vinegar
- 1tsp garlic powder
- 30g butter, cubed

For the slaw:

- 120g blue cheese, crumbled
- 150g soured cream
- 4tbsp mayonnaise
- 1tbsp finely chopped chives
- 1 lemon, juiced
- granny smith apple, cored and cut into matchsticks

- celery, finely chopped
- ¼ medium white cabbage, finely chopped
- pointed spring cabbage, finely chopped

Directions:

Heat the oven to 180C/160C fan/ gas 4. Lay the chicken skin-side up in a roasting tin. Slash the skin of the chicken with a sharp knife, then season and roast for 35 mins. Mix together the hot sauce, paprika, sugar, vinegar, garlic powder and butter in a pan. Stir over a low heat until the butter has melted, then simmer for 1 min. Season. Tip away any excess juices and fat from the roasting tin, then pour in half the sauce. Return to the oven for 20 mins until cooked through. Turn the oven to the highest temperature and add the remaining sauce. Cook for 5 mins. Crumble the cheese into a bowl and mix through the soured cream, mayo, chives and lemon juice. Toss the apple with the celery, cabbage and the cheese sauce. Serve the chicken alongside the slaw.

Nutrition:

Kcal 769, Fat: 64g, Saturates: 21g, Carbs:12g, Sugars: 12g, Fibre: 4g, Protein: 34g, Salt: 2.1g

49. Baked Buffalo Chicken Wings

Preparation Time: 10 mins

Cooking Time: 1 hr

Serves: 12 as a canapé

Ingredients:

- 3 garlic cloves, crushed
- 2 tbsp olive oil
- 3 tbsp cider vinegar
- 1 tbsp paprika
- 1 tbsp Worcestershire sauce
- 2 tsp celery salt
- 4 tbsp pepper sauce
- 3 tbsp honey
- 1 ½kg chicken wing, halved at the joint

Directions:

In a large bowl, mix together the garlic, olive oil, cider vinegar, paprika, Worcestershire sauce, celery salt, hot sauce, honey and a couple of cracks of black pepper. Add the chicken wings and toss around to make sure they're fully covered in the marinade. If you have time, leave the wings to marinate for a couple of hrs in the fridge or ideally overnight. Heat oven to 180C/160C fan/gas 4. Drain and reserve the marinade, then spread the wings out on a very large baking tray. Bake for 30 mins, then pour off the excess oil, add the reserved marinade and toss well. Increase oven to 200C/180C fan/ gas 6. Return to the oven and cook for a further 30 mins, tossing a few times to coat in the glaze as they cook. They should be sticky and glazed with most of the marinade evaporated. Serve on a large platter alongside other party snacks.

Nutrition:
Kcal 210, Fat: 14g, Saturates: 4g, Carbs: 4g, Sugars: 3g, Fibre: 0g, Protein: 17g, Low in salt: 0.94g

50. Buffalo Cauliflower

Preparation Time: 5 mins

Cooking Time: 35 mins

Serves: 4-6 as a starter

Ingredients:

- 1 tbsp sweet smoked paprika
- 1/2 tbsp ground cumin
- 1 tsp garlic powder
- 100g plain flour
- 200ml buttermilk or kefir
- 1 head of cauliflower (500g), broken into florets
- 80g hot sauce
- 1½ tbsp maple syrup
- 1 tbsp butter
- celery sticks, to serve

For the ranch dip:

- 100g Greek yogurt
- 3 tbsp mayonnaise
- 2 tbsp chopped chives
- 1-2 tbsp milk

Directions:

Heat the oven to 220C/200C fan/gas 7 and line a baking tray with baking parchment. Mix together the paprika, cumin, garlic powder, flour and ½ tsp salt in a large bowl. Make a well in the centre and whisk in the buttermilk. Tip in the cauliflower and toss to coat. Spread out the cauliflower on the baking tray and cook for 20-25 mins, turning halfway through, until crisp at the edges. Warm the hot sauce, maple syrup and butter in a small pan set over low heat, for 2-3 mins. Liberally brush over the cauliflower and put back in the oven for 8-10 mins. For the ranch dip, whisk together the yogurt, mayo, chives, milk and a pinch of salt in a bowl. Serve the with the cauliflower alongside some celery sticks for dipping.

Nutrition: Per serving (6)

Kcal 279,	Fat: 17g,	Saturates: 3g,
Carbs: 23g,	Sugars: 9g,	Fibre: 3g,
Protein: 7g,		Salt: 1.1g

51. Pineapple & Pork Skewers

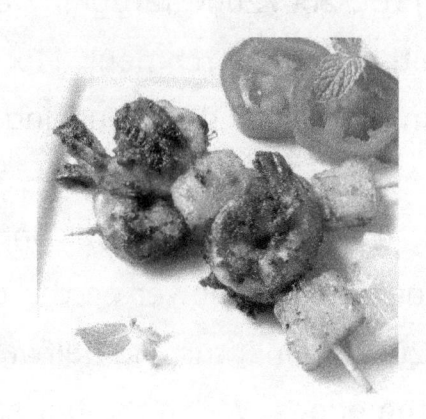

Preparation Time: 20 mins

Cooking Time: 5 mins-10 mins, plus marinating

Serves: 4

Ingredients:

- 400g pork fillet
- 4 tbsp light muscovado sugar
- 60ml cider vinegar
- 1 tsp fish sauce
- ½ small pineapple , peeled, cored and cut into chunks (or use ready prepped fresh pineapple, drained well)
- 1 green pepper , deseeded and cut into squares (optional)

- 4 spring onions , trimmed and cut into 4 equal lengths
- small bunch coriander , chopped (optional)
- cooked rice or pitta, to serve

Directions:

Cut the pork into cubes. Heat the sugar and vinegar in a pan over a low heat until the sugar melts. Add the fish sauce and cool. Tip in the pork and mix well so that all the cubes are covered in sauce. Heat the barbecue. If you are using coals, wait until they turn white. If you are indoors, heat a griddle pan. Thread the pork and pineapple onto skewers, alternating pieces with the pepper and spring onion. Barbecue or griddle the skewers for 3-4 mins each side (you may need to cook them for longer if griddling). Sprinkle with coriander, if you like, then serve with rice or slide into pitta breads.

CHOOSE YOUR SKEWERS:

You'll need eight small or four large skewers for this recipe. Metal skewers with twists along the length are ideal, as they stop the ingredients from sliding about. If you're using wooden skewers, soak them in water first.

Nutrition:

Kcal 260, Fat:7g, Saturates:2g, Salt: 0.4g, Carbs: 26g, Sugars: 26g, Fibre: 2g, Protein: 23g,